MEDITERRANEAN DIET COOKBOOK

THE COMPLETE MEDITERRANEAN DIET GUIDE

By
OKONGOR NDIFON

Copyright © 2023 Okongor Ndifon

Below are Books For Your Delight;

Click On Anyone to Buy or Leave a Review (Thanks a lot).

- <u>ICE CREAM COOKBOOK: HOW TO MAKE ICE CREAM</u>

- <u>25 HEALTHY RECIPES</u>

- <u>**HEALTHY EATING: EAT WELL AND STAY WELL**</u>

- <u>**FLAVORS OF THE WORLD: A CULINARY JOURNEY THROUGH COUNTRIES**</u>

- <u>**RECIPE BOOK PLANNER**</u>

- <u>**DIET JOURNAL**</u>

- <u>**FOOD JOURNAL: FOOD AND FITNESS JOURNAL**</u>

- <u>**MEAL PLANNER LOG BOOK**</u>

- <u>**WEEKLY MEAL PLANNER**</u>

- <u>**RECIPE JOURNAL BOOK**</u>

DISCLAIMER

The book "Mediterranean Diet Cookbook: The Complete Mediterranean Diet Guide" is intended for educational and informational purposes only and should not be considered as legal advice.

DEDICATION

The book, "Mediterranean Diet Cookbook: The Complete Mediterranean Diet Guide", is dedicated to all lovers of good and healthy living.

TABLE OF CONTENTS

1. INTRODUCTION

Embarking on a journey to a healthier lifestyle, Sarah eagerly embraced the "Mediterranean Diet Cookbook."

Its simple yet delectable recipes became her compass, guiding her towards wholesome eating.

The cookbook's easy to follow instructions and vibrant illustrations transformed her kitchen into a haven of fresh ingredients and aromatic herbs.

As she explored the Mediterranean   inspired dishes, Sarah noticed a positive shift in her well being.

The cookbook not only demystified nutritious cooking but also ignited a passion for flavorsome, heart   healthy meals.

 With each recipe, she uncovered the benefits of nourishing her body with the richness of olive oil, vibrant vegetables, and lean proteins.

Sarah's journey wasn't just about food; it was a transformation.

The cookbook became her ally in crafting meals that were not only delicious but also fueled her newfound vitality.

Her story is a testament to the empowering journey one can embark on with the right guide, turning a cookbook into a compass for a healthier, more vibrant life.

Join us on a journey inspired by the transformative experience of Sarah.

Discover how, through the pages of this cookbook, she turned her kitchen into a haven of fresh ingredients and aromatic herbs, not just for meals but for vibrant living.

As we get into simple yet delectable recipes, you're invited to make your kitchen a place of joy, health, and wholesome indulgence.

Benefits of the Mediterranean Diet

Uncover the science backed advantages awaiting you.

From improved heart health to heightened energy levels, we'll see the benefits that make the Mediterranean diet a beacon of well   being.

Sarah's story is a testament to the empowering journey that awaits you as you turn these pages, a journey toward a healthier, more vibrant you.

Here comes the benefits of using Mediterranean diet :

1. Heart Health:
Abundant in heart healthy fats, such as olive oil and omega 3 fatty acids from fish, the Mediterranean diet is associated with a reduced risk of heart disease.

These fats help lower bad cholesterol levels and support cardiovascular health.

2.   Rich in Antioxidants:
The diet is rich in fruits, vegetables, and nuts, providing a plethora of antioxidants.

Antioxidants help combat oxidative stress and inflammation in the body, contributing to a lower risk of chronic diseases.

3.   Improved Weight Management:
 With an emphasis on whole, nutrient   dense foods, the Mediterranean diet supports healthy weight management.

The inclusion of fiber rich foods helps promote satiety, reducing the likelihood of overeating.

4.   Enhanced Cognitive Function:
 The diet's components, such as fatty fish, nuts, and olive oil, have been linked to improved cognitive function and a reduced risk of age related cognitive decline.

Your brain will function better if nourished by nutrients from the Mediterranean diet.

5.   Blood Sugar Control:
 The Mediterranean diet includes whole grains, legumes, and low glycemic fruits, promoting stable blood sugar levels.

This aspect is particularly beneficial for individuals with or at risk of type 2 diabetes.

6.   Inflammation Reduction:
 The anti inflammatory properties of the diet contribute to lowering chronic inflammation in the body.

Chronic inflammation is associated with various diseases, including cardiovascular issues and autoimmune conditions.

7.   Balanced Macronutrients:
 The diet maintains a balance of carbohydrates, proteins, and fats, with an emphasis on healthy fats and lean proteins.

This balanced approach supports overall nutritional needs and energy levels.

8. Gut Health:
 The diet's focus on fiber rich foods, including fruits, vegetables, and whole grains, fosters a healthy gut microbiome.

 A diverse and balanced gut microbiota is linked to improved digestion and immune function.

9. Longevity and Reduced Risk of Chronic Diseases:

 Population studies have consistently shown that adherence to the Mediterranean diet is associated with increased longevity and a decreased risk of chronic diseases, including certain cancers and neurodegenerative conditions.

These science backed benefits collectively make the Mediterranean diet a beacon of well being, offering not just a way of eating but a holistic approach to promoting health and longevity.

2. GETTING STARTED: NAVIGATION THE MEDITERRANEAN KITCHEN

Embarking on your Mediterranean culinary journey begins with understanding the essential ingredients and equipping your kitchen with the right tools.

Let's explore the foundations that will set the stage for your flavorful adventure.

Essential Ingredients in the Mediterranean Diet:

1. Olive Oil:

Often referred to as liquid gold, extra virgin olive oil is a cornerstone of the Mediterranean diet. Rich in monounsaturated fats and antioxidants, it's a versatile and heart healthy choice for cooking and dressing.

2. Fresh Vegetables and Fruits:

Colorful, nutrient packed vegetables and fruits form the basis of Mediterranean meals. From tomatoes and bell peppers to leafy greens and citrus fruits, these provide vitamins, minerals, and antioxidants.

3. Whole Grains:

 Opt for whole grains like quinoa, bulgur, and farro. These grains offer a hearty texture, fiber, and a variety of nutrients, contributing to sustained energy levels.

4. Lean Proteins:

Fish and poultry are preferred sources of protein in the Mediterranean diet. Fatty fish, such as salmon and mackerel, bring omega 3 fatty acids crucial for heart health.

5. Nuts and Seeds:

Almonds, walnuts, and flaxseeds are staples. Packed with healthy fats, proteins, and fiber, they make for nutritious snacks and add a delightful crunch to dishes.

6. Legumes:

Beans, lentils, and chickpeas are excellent plant based protein sources. They are versatile, budget friendly, and contribute to the diet's fiber content.

7. Herbs and Spices:

Elevate your dishes with the aromatic flavors of basil, oregano, rosemary, and garlic. Herbs and spices not only enhance taste but also provide additional health benefits.

Kitchen Tools for Everyone:

1. Quality Chef's Knife:

A sharp, durable chef's knife is your kitchen's workhorse. It facilitates precise chopping and slicing, making meal preparation efficient.

2. Cutting Board:

Invest in a spacious, easy to clean cutting board. Choose materials like bamboo or plastic for durability and hygiene.

3. Vegetable Peeler:

A handy tool for peeling and slicing vegetables, ensuring you can easily incorporate a variety of fresh produce into your meals.

4. Nonstick Pan:

A nonstick pan reduces the need for excessive cooking oils. Ideal for sautéing vegetables, cooking lean proteins, and preparing Mediterranean style dishes.

5. Citrus Juicer:

Extracting fresh juice from lemons or oranges adds a burst of flavor to many Mediterranean recipes. A citrus juicer makes this task a breeze.

With these essential ingredients and friendly kitchen tools, you're poised to dive into the world of Mediterranean cuisine. Let the journey begin

3. BREAKFAST DELIGHTS:RISE AND SHINE WITH MEDITERRANEAN FLAVORS

Mornings set the tone for the day, and with the Mediterranean Diet Cookbook, your breakfast becomes a delightful exploration of flavors and nourishment.

Discover energizing morning recipes and quick, healthy choices that make breakfast a celebration of the Mediterranean lifestyle.

Energizing Morning Recipes:

1. Mediterranean Omelette:
a. Ingredients:
 - 3 large eggs
 - ½ cup diced tomatoes
 - 1 cup fresh spinach, chopped
 - ¼ cup crumbled feta cheese
 - Salt and pepper to taste
 - 1 tablespoon olive oil
 - Fresh herbs for garnish (optional)

b. Instructions:

1. Crack the eggs into a bowl, season with salt and pepper, and whisk until well combined.

2. Heat olive oil in a nonstick pan over medium heat.

3. Add diced tomatoes to the pan and sauté for 2 minutes until slightly softened.

4. Add chopped spinach to the pan and cook until wilted.

5. Pour the whisked eggs over the vegetables in the pan.

6. Allow the eggs to set around the edges, then gently lift and fold with a spatula.

7. Sprinkle crumbled feta cheese over the omelette and continue cooking until the eggs are fully set but still moist.

8. Slide the omelette onto a plate, garnish with fresh herbs if desired, and serve hot.

Enjoy this Mediterranean-inspired omelette for a delicious and nutritious breakfast!

2. Greek Yogurt Parfait:
a. Ingredients:
 - 1 cup Greek yogurt
 - 2 tablespoons honey
 - ¼ cup mixed nuts (almonds, walnuts), chopped
 - ½ cup mixed berries (strawberries, blueberries, raspberries)
 - Garnish with fresh mint leaves (optional).

b. Instructions:
 1. In a bowl, mix Greek yogurt with honey until well combined.

 2. Arrange the Greek yogurt mixture in layers in serving bowls or glasses.

 3. Add a layer of mixed nuts on top of the yogurt.

 4. Follow with a layer of mixed berries.

 5. Continue layering until the bowl or glass is full.

 6. Garnish the top with additional nuts and a drizzle of honey if desired.

 7. Optionally, add fresh mint leaves for a burst of freshness.

 8. Serve immediately and enjoy this wholesome Greek Yogurt Parfait!

This delightful parfait is not only visually appealing but also a nutritious way to start your day or enjoy as a satisfying snack.

3. Whole Grain Pancakes with Berries:
a. Ingredients:
 - 1 cup whole wheat flour
 - 1 tablespoon baking powder
 - 1 tablespoon sugar
 - ½ teaspoon salt
 - 1 cup milk
 - 1 large egg
 - 2 tablespoons olive oil
 - Fresh berries (strawberries, blueberries) for topping
 - Greek yogurt for serving (optional)

b. Instructions:
 1. In a mixing bowl, whisk together whole wheat flour, baking powder, sugar, and salt.

 2. In a separate bowl, beat the egg and then add milk and olive oil. Mix well.

 3. Add the wet mixture to the dry mixture and stir just until blended. It's okay to have some lumps; don't overmix.

 4. Heat a nonstick pan or griddle over medium heat.

5. Pour ¼ cup of batter onto the pan for each pancake.
Continue until the batter is gone.

6. Cook until surface bubbles appear, then turn and cook until golden brown on other side.

7. Continue until the batter is gone.

8. Serve the pancakes topped with fresh berries and, if desired, a dollop of Greek yogurt.

These whole grain pancakes with berries are a delicious and nutritious twist to a classic breakfast favorite.

Enjoy a wholesome start to your day!

4. Avocado Toast with Poached Egg:
a. Ingredients:
 - 1 ripe avocado
 - 2 slices whole grain bread
 - 2 large eggs
 - Salt and pepper to taste
 - Red pepper flakes for garnish (optional)
 - Lemon wedges for serving

b. Instructions:
 1. Toast the slices of whole grain bread to your desired level of crispiness.

2. While the bread is toasting, scoop out the ripe avocado and mash it in a bowl. Add salt and pepper to taste.

3. Spread the mashed avocado evenly over the toasted bread slices.

4. Simmer some water in a shallow pan. Add a splash of vinegar.

5. Crack each egg into a small bowl and gently slide them into the simmering water.

6. Poach the eggs for about 3-4 minutes until the whites are set but the yolks are still runny.

7. Using a slotted spoon, carefully place one poached egg on each avocado-covered toast.

8. Sprinkle with additional salt, pepper, and red pepper flakes if desired.

9. Serve immediately with lemon wedges on the side for an extra burst of freshness.

This Avocado Toast with Poached Egg is a savory and satisfying breakfast that combines creamy avocado with the perfect runniness of a poached egg.

Savor a wholesome and delectable way to begin the day!

Quick and Healthy Breakfast Choices:

1.   Mediterranean Smoothie Bowl:
a.   Ingredients:
   - 1 cup of frozen mixed berries, including raspberries, blueberries, and strawberries
   - 1 ripe banana, frozen
   - ½ cup Greek yogurt
   - 1 tablespoon olive oil
   - ¼ cup granola
   - 1 tablespoon chia seeds
   - Fresh mint leaves for garnish
   - Honey for drizzling (optional)

b.   Instructions:
   1. In a blender, combine frozen berries, frozen banana, Greek yogurt, and olive oil.

   2. Blend until smooth and creamy, adding a splash of water or milk if needed to reach your desired consistency.

   3. Transfer the blended drink to a bowl.

   4. Top the smoothie with granola, chia seeds, and fresh mint leaves.

5. Drizzle with honey if you prefer an extra touch of sweetness.

6. Customize your bowl with additional toppings like sliced almonds or coconut flakes if desired.

7. Serve immediately and enjoy this refreshing and nutrient-packed Mediterranean Smoothie Bowl!

This vibrant and nourishing smoothie bowl is a delightful way to infuse your mornings with Mediterranean goodness.

Suck into a bowl full of flavor and freshness!

2. Muesli with Fresh Fruit:
a.   Ingredients:
  - 1 cup rolled oats
  - 1 cup Greek yogurt
  - 1 cup of milk (vegan or dairy).
  - 1 tablespoon honey
  - ¼ cup mixed nuts (almonds, walnuts), chopped
  - ½ cup mixed dried fruits (figs, dates, apricots), chopped
  - Fresh fruits (berries, banana slices) for topping

b.   Instructions:

1. In a mixing bowl, combine rolled oats, Greek yogurt, milk, and honey. Stir until well mixed.

2. Cover the bowl and refrigerate the mixture overnight or for at least 4 hours to allow the oats to soften.

3. Before serving, give the muesli a good stir. If necessary, thin the consistency with more milk.

4. Mix in chopped nuts and dried fruits.

5. Spoon the muesli into serving bowls.

6. Top each bowl with fresh fruits of your choice.

7. Optionally, drizzle with an extra swirl of honey for sweetness.

8. Serve chilled and savor the wholesome goodness of this Muesli with Fresh Fruit!

This make-ahead muesli is a convenient and nutritious breakfast option, perfect for busy mornings or as a refreshing snack.

Savor the delicious fusion of flavors and textures!

3. Mediterranean Breakfast Wrap:

a.   **Ingredients:**
   - 1 whole wheat wrap or tortilla
   - 2 tablespoons hummus
   - ½ cup cherry tomatoes, halved
   - ¼ cucumber, thinly sliced
   - ¼ cup feta cheese, crumbled
   - Fresh spinach leaves
   - Kalamata olives, sliced (optional)
   - Olive oil for drizzling
   - Salt and pepper to taste

b.   **Instructions:**

1. Lay the whole wheat wrap on a flat surface.

2. Spread a layer of hummus over the entire surface of the wrap.

3. Arrange a handful of fresh spinach leaves in the center of the wrap.

4. Add halved cherry tomatoes, thinly sliced cucumber, and crumbled feta cheese on top of the spinach.

5. If desired, sprinkle sliced Kalamata olives over the ingredients.

6. Drizzle olive oil over the filling, and season with salt and pepper to taste.

7. Fold in the sides of the wrap and then roll it tightly, creating a burrito-style wrap.

8. Slice the wrap in half diagonally for easy serving.

This Mediterranean Breakfast Wrap offers a delightful combination of flavors and textures, making it a perfect portable breakfast or a quick and healthy lunch option.

Enjoy the Mediterranean goodness in every bite!

4. Fruit and Nut Breakfast Couscous:

a.   Ingredients:
  - 1 cup couscous
  - 1 ½ cups water
  - ¼ cup dried fruits (apricots, cranberries), chopped
  - 2 tablespoons mixed nuts (almonds, pistachios), chopped
  - 1 tablespoon honey
  - ½ teaspoon cinnamon
  - Greek yogurt for serving (optional)

b.   Instructions:

1. Boil some water in a saucepan.

2. Stir in couscous, cover, and remove from heat. Let it sit for 5 minutes or until the couscous absorbs the water.

3. Use a fork to separate the grains in the couscous.

4. Add chopped dried fruits and mixed nuts to the couscous, mixing well.

5. Drizzle honey over the mixture and sprinkle with cinnamon. Stir until evenly distributed.

6. If desired, serve the breakfast couscous over a bed of Greek yogurt.

7. Optionally, garnish with additional nuts and a drizzle of honey for extra indulgence.

8. Enjoy this delightful Fruit and Nut Breakfast Couscous as a satisfying and nutritious way to start your day!

This couscous dish offers a unique twist to your morning routine, combining the wholesome goodness of fruits and nuts for a flavorful breakfast experience.

Start your day with these breakfast delights that not only tantalize your taste buds but also infuse your morning with the vitality of Mediterranean goodness.

Breakfast has never been this deliciously healthy!

4. FRESH AND VIBRANT SALADS

4.1 Simple Salad Creations

Recipe: Greek Salad

a. Ingredients:
- 2 cups cherry tomatoes, halved
- 1 cucumber, diced
- 1 red onion, thinly sliced
- 1 cup Kalamata olives, pitted
- 1 cup feta cheese, crumbled
- 1/4 cup extra-virgin olive oil
- 2 tablespoons red non alcoholic wine vinegar
- 1 teaspoon dried oregano
- Salt and pepper to taste

b. Instructions:
1. Cherry tomatoes, cucumber, red onion, olives, and feta cheese should all be combined in a big bowl.

2. Combine the olive oil, non alcoholic wine, vinegar, dried oregano, salt, and pepper in a small bowl.

3. After adding the dressing to the salad, gently toss to coat all of the ingredients.

4. Allow the salad to marinate in the refrigerator for at least 30 minutes before serving.

5. Serve chilled and enjoy the refreshing flavors of this classic Greek salad.

4.2 Dressings for Flavorful Salads

Recipe: Lemon-Herb Vinaigrette

a. Ingredients:
- 1/3 cup extra-virgin olive oil
- 2 tablespoons fresh lemon juice
- 1 teaspoon Dijon mustard
- 1 clove garlic, minced
- 1 tablespoon fresh parsley, chopped
- Salt and pepper to taste

b. Instructions:
1. In a small bowl, whisk together olive oil, lemon juice, Dijon mustard, minced garlic, and chopped parsley.

2. Season with salt and pepper to taste, adjusting the quantities based on your preference.

3. Whisk until the dressing is well emulsified.

4. Drizzle the lemon-herb vinaigrette over your favorite salad just before serving.

5. Toss gently to ensure every leaf is coated, enhancing your salad with a burst of citrusy freshness.

These simple recipes will add a Mediterranean flair to your salads, making them a delightful addition to your culinary repertoire.

5. WHOLESOME SOUPS AND STEWS

5.1 Hearty Mediterranean Soups

Recipe: Minestrone Soup

a.   Ingredients:
- 2 tablespoons olive oil
- 1 onion, diced
- 2 carrots, chopped
- 2 celery stalks, diced
- 3 cloves garlic, minced
- 1 14-oz can of diced tomatoes
- 1 15 ounces can of rinsed and drained cannellini beans
- 4 cups vegetable broth
- - A single cup of tiny pasta, like ditalini
- 1 teaspoon dried basil
- 1 teaspoon dried oregano
- Salt and pepper to taste
- Freshly grated Parmesan for serving

b.   Instructions:
1. Heat the olive oil in a big pot over medium heat.

Add onion, carrots, celery, and garlic.

Sauté until vegetables are softened.

2. Stir in diced tomatoes, cannellini beans, vegetable broth, pasta, basil, oregano, salt, and pepper.

3. Bring the soup to a boil, then reduce heat and simmer for 15-20 minutes or until pasta is tender.

4. Serve hot, garnished with freshly grated Parmesan.

5.2 Nourishing Stews for Everyone

Recipe: Mediterranean Chickpea Stew

a. Ingredients:
- 2 tablespoons olive oil
- 1 onion, finely chopped
- 2 carrots, sliced
- 2 cloves garlic, minced
– A single 15-oz can of rinsed and drained chickpeas
- A single 14-oz can of diced tomatoes
- 1 cup vegetable broth
- 1 teaspoon ground cumin
- 1 teaspoon smoked paprika
- Salt and pepper to taste

- Fresh parsley for garnish

b. Instructions:
 1. Heat the olive oil in a big pot over medium heat.

Add chopped onion, carrots, and garlic.

Sauté until onions are translucent.

 2. Add chickpeas, diced tomatoes, vegetable broth, cumin, smoked paprika, salt, and pepper.

 3. Bring the stew to a simmer, then cover and cook for 20-25 minutes.

 4. Adjust seasoning if needed and serve hot, garnished with fresh parsley.

These hearty soups and stews capture the essence of the Mediterranean, offering warmth and nourishment for both body and soul. Enjoy the comforting flavors of these friendly recipes.

6. DELECTABLE MAIN DISHES

6.1 Easy-to-Make Mediterranean Entrées

Recipe: Lemon Herb Chicken Skewers

a.   Ingredients:
 - 1.5 pounds of chopped, skinless, boneless chicken breasts
 - 1/4 cup olive oil
 - 3 tablespoons fresh lemon juice
 - 2 cloves garlic, minced
 - 1 teaspoon dried oregano
 - 1 teaspoon dried thyme
 - Salt and pepper to taste
 - Wooden skewers, soaked in water

b.   Instructions:
 1. In a bowl, whisk together olive oil, lemon juice, minced garlic, oregano, thyme, salt, and pepper.

 2. For at least half an hour, marinate the chicken chunks in the mixture.

 3. Preheat the grill or grill pan over medium-high heat.

4. Thread marinated chicken onto the soaked skewers.

5. Grill skewers for 6-8 minutes, turning occasionally until chicken is cooked through.

6. Serve hot with your favorite Mediterranean side dishes.

6.2 Seafood, Poultry, and Vegetarian Options

Recipe: Mediterranean Quinoa Bowl

a.   Ingredients:
- 1 cup quinoa, rinsed
- 2 cups water or vegetable broth
- 1 tablespoon olive oil
- 1 onion, finely chopped
- 2 sliced bell peppers of various colors
- 1 zucchini, diced
- 1 cup cherry tomatoes, halved
- A single 15-oz can of rinsed and drained chickpeas
- 1 teaspoon ground cumin
- 1 teaspoon smoked paprika
- Salt and pepper to taste
- Feta cheese for garnish (optional)
- Fresh parsley for garnish

b.   Instructions:
1. In a saucepan, combine quinoa and water or broth.

After bringing to a boil, lower the heat, cover, and simmer the quinoa for 15 to 20 minutes, or until it is tender.

2. In a large skillet, heat olive oil over medium heat.

Add chopped onion, bell peppers, and zucchini. Sauté until vegetables are tender.

3. Stir in cherry tomatoes, chickpeas, cumin, smoked paprika, salt, and pepper.

Cook for an additional 5 minutes.

4. Serve the vegetable mixture over cooked quinoa, garnished with feta cheese (if desired) and fresh parsley.

These easy-to-make Mediterranean entrées showcase the diverse flavors of the region, catering to seafood lovers, poultry enthusiasts, and those embracing a vegetarian lifestyle.

Enjoy these delightful main dishes that bring the essence of the Mediterranean to your table.

7. SIDES AND SNACKS

7.1 Tasty Bites for Any Occasion

Recipe: Mediterranean Hummus Platter

a.   Ingredients:
– A single 15-oz can of rinsed and drained chickpeas
- 1/4 cup tahini
- 3 tablespoons extra-virgin olive oil
- 2 cloves garlic, minced
- Juice of 1 lemon
- 1/2 teaspoon ground cumin
- Salt and pepper to taste
- Assorted veggies (carrot sticks, cucumber slices, cherry tomatoes) for dipping
- Pita bread, cut into wedges

b.   Instructions:
1. In a food processor, combine chickpeas, tahini, olive oil, minced garlic, lemon juice, cumin, salt, and pepper.

2. Blend until smooth, adding water if needed to reach your desired consistency.

3. Transfer the hummus to a serving platter.

4. Arrange assorted veggies and pita wedges around the hummus.

5. Serve as a delightful and flavorful appetizer for any occasion.

7.2 Nutrient-Packed Side Dishes

Recipe: Roasted Mediterranean Vegetables

a.   Ingredients:
- 2 cups cherry tomatoes, halved
- 1 zucchini, sliced
- 1 yellow bell pepper, sliced
- 1 red onion, thinly sliced
- 2 tablespoons olive oil
- 1 teaspoon dried oregano
- 1 teaspoon dried thyme
- Salt and pepper to taste
- Feta cheese for garnish (optional)
- Fresh basil for garnish

b.   Instructions:

1. Set oven temperature to 400°F, or 200°C.

2. In a large bowl, toss cherry tomatoes, zucchini, bell pepper, and red onion with olive oil, oregano, thyme, salt, and pepper.

3. Arrange the veggies in a single layer on a baking sheet.

4. Roast the vegetables for 20 to 25 minutes, or until they are soft and have taken on a hint of caramel.

5. Garnish with crumbled feta cheese (if desired) and fresh basil before serving.

These tasty bites and nutrient-packed side dishes complement any Mediterranean meal, providing a perfect balance of flavors and textures for your culinary enjoyment.

Incorporate these recipes into your repertoire for delightful snacks and accompaniments.

8. SWEET ENDINGS

8.1 Mediterranean-inspired Desserts

Recipe: Orange and Almond Cake

a.   Ingredients:
- 1 cup almond flour
- 1 cup sugar
- 4 large eggs
- Zest of 2 oranges
- Juice of 1 orange
- 1 teaspoon baking powder
- 1/2 teaspoon vanilla extract
- Powdered sugar for dusting (optional)
- Orange slices for garnish

b.   Instructions:
1. Preheat the oven to 350°F (180°C). Grease and line a cake pan.

2. In a bowl, whisk together almond flour, sugar, eggs, orange zest, orange juice, baking powder, and vanilla extract until well combined.

3. Pour the batter into the prepared pan and bake for 30-35 minutes or until a toothpick inserted comes out clean.

4. After letting the cake cool in the pan for ten minutes, move it to a wire rack to finish cooling.

5. Dust with powdered sugar (if desired) and garnish with orange slices before serving.

8.2 Guilt-Free Treats for Everyone

Recipe: Greek Yogurt and Honey Parfait

a.   Ingredients:
  - 1 cup Greek yogurt
  - 2 tablespoons honey
  - 1/2 cup of mixed berries, including raspberries, blueberries, and strawberries
  - 2 tablespoons of finely chopped nuts (walnuts, almonds)
  - Fresh mint leaves for garnish

b.   Instructions:
  1. In a glass or bowl, layer Greek yogurt, drizzle with honey, and add a handful of mixed berries.

  2. Repeat the layers until you reach the top, finishing with a drizzle of honey and a sprinkle of chopped nuts.

  3. Garnish with fresh mint leaves.

4. Serve immediately for a refreshing and guilt-
free dessert.

These Mediterranean-inspired desserts offer a
delightful conclusion to your meals.

Enjoy the rich flavors of the Orange and Almond
Cake or savor the freshness of the Greek Yogurt
and Honey Parfait—guilt-free treats that capture the
essence of the Mediterranean sweet experience.

9. TIPS FOR SUCCESS

9.1 Meal Planning for Everyone

Embarking on the Mediterranean diet journey involves thoughtful meal planning to ensure a seamless and enjoyable experience.

Here are some tips:

- **Diverse Ingredients:**

Embrace a variety of colorful fruits, vegetables, whole grains, and lean proteins.

Incorporate different textures and flavors to keep your meals interesting.

- **Weekly Menu:**

Plan your meals for the week, considering your schedule and preferences.

This helps streamline grocery shopping and reduces the chances of opting for less healthy alternatives.

-        **Batch Cooking:**

Prepare larger quantities of key components like grains, roasted vegetables, or protein sources.

 This makes assembling meals during the week quick and convenient.

-        **Seasonal Choices:**

 Choose seasonal produce for freshness and cost-effectiveness.

It ensures that your meals align with the flavors traditionally associated with the Mediterranean diet.

9.2 Incorporating Mediterranean Habits into Daily Life

Making the Mediterranean diet a lifestyle involves more than just meal choices. Here are practical tips for seamlessly incorporating Mediterranean habits into your daily routine:

- **Active Lifestyle:**

Embrace a more active lifestyle by incorporating daily walks, bike rides, or engaging in outdoor activities.

An essential component of the Mediterranean lifestyle is physical activity.

- **Social Meals:**

Share meals with friends and family.

The Mediterranean tradition values the communal aspect of dining, fostering a sense of connection and enjoyment.

- **Mindful Eating:**

Slow down and savor each bite.

Take note of your food's flavors and textures. Eating with awareness improves the whole dining experience.

This mindful approach to eating enhances the overall dining experience.

- **Hydration with Water and Herbs:**

Replace sugary drinks with water infused with fresh herbs like mint or basil.

Hydration is crucial, and this habit adds a refreshing twist to your daily water intake.

By incorporating these meal planning strategies and lifestyle habits, you can seamlessly adopt the Mediterranean way of living, promoting both physical and mental well-being.

Enjoy the journey as you cultivate a healthier and more flavorful lifestyle.

10. CONCLUSION

Congratulations on completing your culinary
journey into Mediterranean cooking!

As you reflect on the pages of this friendly
cookbook, filled with vibrant recipes and practical
tips, take a moment to celebrate the progress
you've made.

Embracing the Mediterranean lifestyle is not just
about the food on your plate; it's a holistic approach
to well-being.

The flavorful dishes, rich in fruits, vegetables, whole
grains, and lean proteins, are not just recipes but
gateways to a healthier and more enjoyable life.

In your exploration, you've discovered the art of
crafting simple salads, hearty soups, delectable
main dishes, and sweet treats that tantalize the
taste buds while nourishing the body.

Each recipe has been designed to introduce you to
the diverse and delightful flavors of the
Mediterranean.

Beyond the kitchen, you've learned the importance
of meal planning, incorporating seasonal choices,
and adopting a mindful and active lifestyle.

These habits not only enhance your culinary
experience but also contribute to a wholesome way
of life.

As you continue on this journey, remember that the Mediterranean lifestyle is a celebration of good food, shared moments, and a sense of well-being.

Cherish the joy of preparing and sharing these meals with loved ones, savoring each bite, and creating memories around the table.

May your Mediterranean cooking adventure bring fulfillment, health, and a deeper appreciation for the richness of this culinary tradition.

Here's to celebrating your journey and the delightful flavors that will continue to grace your kitchen for years to come.

Buon Appetito

"Enjoy your meal!"

GLOSSARY OF TERMS

1. Mediterranean Diet: A dietary pattern inspired by the traditional eating habits of countries bordering the Mediterranean Sea.

 It emphasizes fruits, vegetables, whole grains, fish, and olive oil while limiting red meat and processed foods.

2. Tzatziki: A Greek condiment made with yogurt, cucumbers, garlic, and herbs.

3. Panzanella: An Italian bread salad typically made with day-old bread, tomatoes, cucumbers, and fresh herbs, drizzled with olive oil.

4. Vinaigrette: A dressing made from a mixture of oil, vinegar, and seasonings, often used to enhance the flavors of salads.

5. Emulsify: The process of combining two liquids, like oil and vinegar, into a stable mixture, as in the preparation of salad dressings.

6.   Ditalini: A type of small pasta, often used in soups and salads, resembling short tubes or small macaroni.

7.   Cannellini Beans: White kidney beans popular in Mediterranean cuisine, known for their creamy texture and mild flavor.

8.   Paprika: A spice made from dried and ground peppers, adding a rich, sweet, or smoky flavor to dishes.

9.   Pita Bread: A round, flatbread common in Mediterranean and Middle Eastern cuisines, often used for dipping or as a base for sandwiches.

10.   Mint Infusion: Water infused with fresh mint leaves, a popular and refreshing alternative to sugary beverages.

11.   Comprehensive Meal Planning: A systematic approach to organizing meals for a week, taking into account nutritional balance, variety, and personal preferences.

12.   Mindful Eating: A practice that involves paying full attention to the sensory experience of eating, promoting a healthier relationship with food.
13.   Minestrone Soup: An Italian vegetable soup with a base of broth, tomatoes, beans, and pasta or rice, often including a variety of seasonal vegetables.

14.   Cumin: A spice with a warm and earthy flavor commonly used in Mediterranean cuisine, adding depth to dishes.

15.   Parsley: A versatile herb used as a garnish or ingredient in Mediterranean recipes, providing a fresh and bright flavor.

16.   Feta Cheese: A tangy and crumbly cheese originating from Greece, commonly used in salads, pastries, and as a topping.

17.   Dijon Mustard: A type of mustard originating from the city of Dijon in France, known for its smooth texture and slightly spicy flavor, often used in dressings and marinades.

18.   Mediterranean Chickpea Stew: A hearty dish made with chickpeas, tomatoes, and a blend of Mediterranean spices, offering a nutritious and flavorful meal.

19.   Caramelization: The process of browning sugars in vegetables or fruits during cooking, enhancing their sweetness and depth of flavor.

20.   Almond Flour: Ground almonds used as a gluten-free alternative in baking, contributing a nutty flavor and moist texture to dishes.

21. Hydration with Herbs: Infusing water with herbs like mint or basil, providing a flavorful and refreshing way to stay hydrated.

22. Communal Dining: A cultural practice emphasizing the social aspect of sharing meals with family and friends, common in Mediterranean traditions.

23. Buon Appetito: An Italian phrase expressing good wishes for a delicious meal, often used as a friendly invitation to enjoy the food.

24. Batter: A mixture typically made from flour, liquid, and other ingredients, used as a base for various dishes, including pancakes, fritters, and certain desserts.

This glossary provides key terms relevant to Mediterranean cooking, helping you navigate the diverse and flavorful world of this culinary tradition.

ABOUT THE AUTHOR

Meet a culinary enthusiast, and passionate advocate for the Mediterranean way of life.

With a background deeply rooted in a love for wholesome, flavorful meals, Okongor Ndifon brings a unique blend of expertise and personal experience to the world of culinary exploration.

Having immersed in the vibrant cultures of the Mediterranean, discovered the transformative power of embracing a diet that not only tantalizes the taste buds but also nourishes the body and soul.

The inspiration to share the joys of Mediterranean cooking led Okongor Ndifon to create this cookbook, weaving together a tapestry of recipes, practical tips, and cultural insights.

Okongor Ndifon believes that cooking is more than a chore; it's a celebration.

Their approach combines a deep appreciation for traditional flavors with a practical understanding of the challenges faced by those just starting their culinary journey.

This commitment to inclusivity and a love for sharing the Mediterranean lifestyle is evident in every page of the cookbook.

As you embark on your culinary adventure through the pages of "Mediterranean Diet Cookbook," consider Okongor Ndifon, your trusted guide, encouraging you to savor the flavors, embrace the habits, and celebrate the joy of cooking.

"HAPPY EATING"